YOUR KNOWLEDGE HAS VALUE

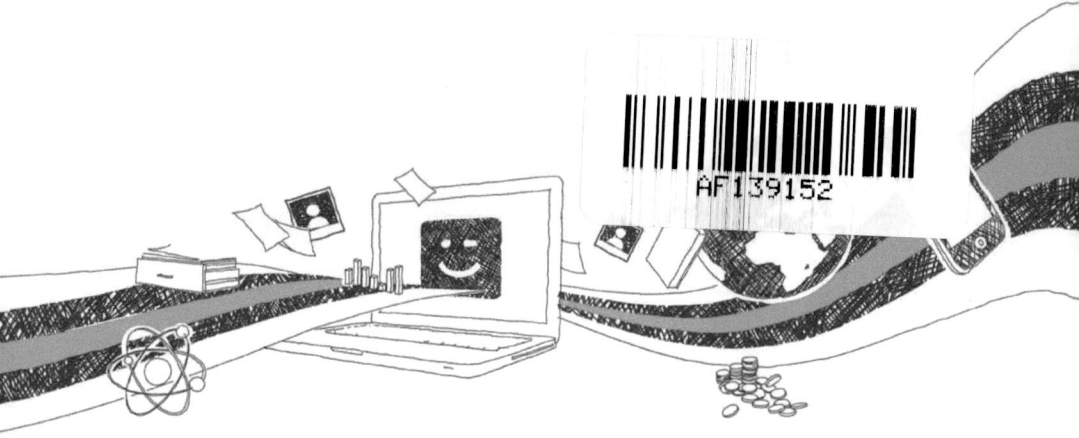

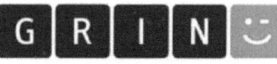

Bibliographic information published by the German National Library:

The German National Library lists this publication in the National Bibliography; detailed bibliographic data are available on the Internet at http://dnb.dnb.de .

Imprint:

Copyright © 2016 GRIN Verlag, Open Publishing GmbH
Print and binding: Books on Demand GmbH, Norderstedt Germany
ISBN: 9783668583252

Patrick Kimuyu

The Affordable Health Care Act (ObamaCare) and the Concept of Universal Healthcare

GRIN Publishing

GRIN - Your knowledge has value

Since its foundation in 1998, GRIN has specialized in publishing academic texts by students, college teachers and other academics as e-book and printed book. The website www.grin.com is an ideal platform for presenting term papers, final papers, scientific essays, dissertations and specialist books.

Visit us on the internet:

http://www.grin.com/

http://www.facebook.com/grincom

http://www.twitter.com/grin_com

Affordable Health Care Act (Obamacare)

Name: Patrick K. Kimuyu

Inhaltsverzeichnis

Abstract.. 3

Introduction 5

   Context: U.S Interest in Universal Healthcare 6

   Methods 7

   Dominant Policy: Universal Health as a Reliable Public Policy 8

   Significance of the Affordable Care Act to the U.S Public... 8

   Impact of Affordable Care Act 11

   Impact of Healthcare Policy Changes to Utilization.. 12

   Policy Counter: Alternative Policy to ObamaCare 13

   Discussion.. 13

Conclusion... 15

References 16

Abstract

Healthcare reforms in the United States have always been faced with challenges, ranging from the drafting of the concerned policies to their implementation. This is probably the reason as to why the U.S healthcare system has never attained remarkable sustainability, especially through the elimination of health inequalities with the population.

However, ObamaCare has attracted unprecedented political criticism, owing to its cost consequences. Therefore, this paper will provide an overview of the U.S context, in which the Affordable Care Act has attracted political criticism. It will also present the methods used to analyze different perspectives of the issue in regard to political narrative strategies, in which the dominant perspective will discuss the concept on universal healthcare as a reliable public policy.

The context presents the concept of universal healthcare provided under the Affordable Care Act, and it explains the challenges faced in establishing reliable healthcare policy reforms over the past four decades.

Methods used in this analysis, primarily the policy change theory presents political narrative strategies as the most relevant approaches for reviewing ObamaCare through a political lens.

For the purpose of analysis, the concept of universal healthcare as a reliable public policy is discussed as the dominant policy in which its impacts are reviewed from various perspectives. On the other hand, alternative policy is discussed as the counter policy in which various approaches are explained to justify its significance in addressing cost issues in the U.S healthcare system.

The discussion provides a comprehensive evaluation of the two policy changes to ascertain the most relevant approach. It also establishes political connections to ObamaCare and its consequences.

Conclusively, ObamaCare serves as an ideal public policy because it will solve insurance problems in healthcare. However, its high cost compromise healthcare sustainability and national economic development.

Policy Problem: Politics of ObamaCare as a public policy

Approach to Analysis: Political narrative strategies

Approach to Research: Literature review, government publications and media reports

Introduction

Healthcare reforms in the United States have always been faced with challenges, ranging from the drafting of the policy concerns to their implementation. This is probably the reason as to why the U.S healthcare system has never attained remarkable sustainability, especially through the elimination of health inequalities with in the population. As a result, healthcare policy changes have become highly politicized in which some political personalities, as well as groups seeking to achieve their political motives through politically instigated policy reforms. For instance, different U.S presidents have attempted to introduce healthcare policy changes to realize universal healthcare, but in vain. However, the Obama Administration seems to have overcome all the challenges faced in the last 40 years in establishing the Affordable Care Act after the unanimous approval by the House of Representatives on March 21, 2010 (GPO, 2009). It is believed that, the quest for the introduction of healthcare reform was occasioned by the inefficiency of the old healthcare system in which access to healthcare services by U.S citizens was somehow difficult. In the old healthcare system, only some few selected groups were able to access healthcare services under Government-funded healthcare program. Healthcare coverage involved Medicare and Medicaid, Government-funded healthcare program through which the elderly and the low-income populations could access medical services in public healthcare institutions.

However, it is worth noting that ObamaCare has become one of the highly politicized public policies. Therefore, a comprehensive review of the Affordable Care Act through a political lens appears relevant to ascertain its significance to U.S citizens.

This paper begins with an overview of the U.S context, in which the Affordable Care Act has attracted political criticism. It will also present the methods used to analyze different perspectives of the issue in regard to political narrative strategies, in which the dominant

5

perspective will discuss the concept on universal healthcare as a reliable public policy. The counter perspective will review the alternative to ObamaCare and the politics surrounding the policy. Finally, the conclusion will provide a summary of the policy change theory under a political lens.

Context: U.S Interest in Universal Healthcare

The U.S healthcare reform is an issue, which has been discussed in an array of articles, although different authors address the topic from diverse perspectives. Cohen (2012) states, "Health care rationing has been a source of contentious debate in the United States for nearly 30 years" (p. 90). On the other hand, Cudney explains that the U.S healthcare system has remained inefficient because; its fragmented structure allows the multiplication of errors (Cudney, 2002).

However, it is worth noting that, the realization of sustainable healthcare has been a dream for U.S citizens because; efficient healthcare reforms were entirely missing. Nevertheless, the Patient Protection and Affordable Care Act appear reliable for the realization of healthcare sustainability in a foreseeable future. APHA (2012) reports, "the law contains hundreds of provisions meant to increase access to health coverage and care, provide a new focus on prevention and public health, bolster the country's health workforce and infrastructure, promote innovation and quality, and control rising health care costs" (p. 1).

This is under federal jurisdiction, in which the U.S health insurance is based on federally-funded programs. Ordinarily, The Federally-funded healthcare programs require individuals to pay the so-called 'deductibles' to supplement their total contributions paid through regular premiums. In contrast, the recent healthcare reforms have created a universal healthcare coverage to all individuals.

Despite the benefits of the Affordable Care Act, different sources have been presenting different perspectives, especially with the accrued benefits of the law. For instance, Blumberg and colleagues argues that the ACA reform will not have a significant impact on employer-sponsored insurance because; most workers will rely on it as a primary source of healthcare coverage. They estimate, "the Affordable Care Act (ACA) will leave employer-sponsored coverage largely intact; in contrast, some economists and benefit consultants argue that the ACA encourages employers to drop coverage, thereby making both their workers and their firms better off" (Blumberg et. al, 2012 p. 116). On the other hand, Goody, Mentnech and Riley (2002) evaluated the changing nature of private and public healthcare insurance and explain the gaps in insurance coverage. They reported, "A mix of public and private solutions such as tax credits for low-income uninsured and Federal funding for State high-risk pools are currently being proposed to make private health insurance more accessible and affordable" (p. 1).

Methods

It is evident that the Affordable Care Act has introduced drastic changes in the U.S healthcare system. However, the scope of the policy is subjective to political reality. Therefore, policy change theory, primarily the use of political narrative strategies seems relevant in reviewing ObamaCare through a political lens.

For the purpose of political narrative strategies, literature related to the topic will provide historical insight and help in unearthing the significance of the policy U.S citizens. Precisely, media reports and transcripts of debates on healthcare reforms will be analyzed to justify the authenticity of the concerned approaches into the matter. In addition, government publications such as the amendments on H.R 3590 draft which addresses the Patient Protection and Affordable Care Act will be used extensively in the policy review (HHS, 2009).

Dominant Policy: Universal Health as a Reliable Public Policy

Universal healthcare entails unlimited access to healthcare services by all U.S citizens, irrespective of gender, age and financial status of the individuals. In practice, universal healthcare is a gateway to improved living standards; since it will guarantee the well-being of all individuals. Sec. 1Title I (Subtitle A) defines how ACA will provide "immediate improvements in health care coverage for all Americans" (HHS 18). It is also intended to reduce the cost of healthcare across the country.

Concisely, universal healthcare is more or less the same as the current Medicaid healthcare program designed for the low-income individuals. In the recent healthcare reforms, all U.S citizens are intended to be eligible for Medicaid benefits irrespective of their ability to pay for the insurance coverage to facilitate access to medical services by all individuals. It is a form of a single-payer system, whereby all individuals will be accorded healthcare insurance coverage equally.

Significance of the Affordable Care Act to the U.S Public

In theory, the Affordable Care Act will benefit various Americans in several ways and introduce universal care with the assistance of several controls and policies. The ACA will benefit different Americans by increasing the quality, affordability and accessibility of care and eliminating discriminatory exclusions. It will attempt to introduce universal care with the assistance of those steps, which can extend coverage to those areas of the population which previously found it hard to have access to care. According to historical research, the ACA will accomplish this by providing a "great opportunity to expand coverage and access, and bring spiraling health care costs under control" (Gorin & Moniz, 2012 p. 195). It is believed that, ObamaCare will address the old-age problem of healthcare insurance and patients' protection. Currently, there are about 48 million uninsured people, in the United States, which translates to

16.3% of the total U.S population. It is surprising that the U.S is one of the wealthiest industrialized nations in the world but, it does not have a universal healthcare system, which involves national health insurance and, this has led to numerous healthcare consequences (Carmen, Proctor & Smith, 2012).

An aesthetic review of insurance coverage indicates that, in 2010, insurance coverage was found to be 83.7 percent of national concern, although the U.S Government-funded insurance program; Medicare, Medicaid and Children's Health Insurance Program accounted for only 31.0%. The remaining coverage percentage was provided by employment-based and direct-purchase insurance, in which they accounted for 55.3% and 9.8% respectively. However, healthcare reports indicate that there was a significant decrease of insured Americans among the U.S population, in 2011. In 2011, the total number of the uninsured population was found to have decreased to 48.6 million and, this was equivalent to 15.7 percent. From an analytical perspective, there was remarkable progress in insurance coverage, in 2011 compared to 2010 in which the total number of the uninsured was 50 million. Consequently, these changes in insurance coverage were reflected on the total number of insured population, in which it increased from 256.6 million, in 2010 to 260.2 million, in 2011 (Carmen, Proctor & Smith, 2012). Ordinarily, there are different health insurance providers, in the United States, these insurance providers can be categorized into two broad groups; the U.S Government-funded health insurance and private health insurance. Government-funded health insurance comprises of Medicaid, Medicare, the veteran and children's health insurance programs, they provide insurance coverage to about 99.5 million people who are among the insured population.

On the other hand, private insurance provides insurance coverage to the largest number of the insured population, and it has been the leading health insurance provider over the past three decades. In 2011, the number of people who were insured under private health insurance was 197.3 million but, this number seems to have remained constant for the last three years, owing to the introduction of healthcare reforms, which have enhanced enrollment of the public into the Government-funded health insurance programs. As a result, the total number of insured people under the government insurance programs increased from 31.2%, in 2010 to 32.2% by the end of 2011, and this percentage is believed to have increased further, in 2012. In regard to the distribution of insurance coverage, the number of insured Americans under employment-based health insurance was 170.1 million, in 2011 and this was equivalent to 55.1 percent of the total percentage of the insured Americans in the United States. Private health insurance coverage was 63.9%, whereas direct-purchase health insurance accounted for 9.8% by 2011 (Carmen, Proctor & Smith, 2012).

However, the observed insurance challenges will be addressed appropriately by the Affordable Care Act. The Center for Medicare and Medicaid Services states that, the Affordable Care Act will offer the U.S population with health security through enhancing efficient healthcare reforms by lowering healthcare costs, ensuring accountability of health insurance companies, expanding healthcare insurance coverage and promoting quality healthcare for all Americans. Therefore, the ACA seems to be a reliable approach, which will grant all Americans with efficient healthcare services; thus, transforming it into a fundamental universal right (Record, 2012).

Impact of Affordable Care Act

In general, the recent healthcare measures have expanded access to healthcare through a number of meaningful ways. For instance, the Affordable Care Act enables young Americans in the U.S workforce to access healthcare under their parent's healthcare plans. In addition, the recent reforms require insurers to offer medical cover to children with existing medical conditions; contrary to the case before in the old healthcare plans in which such individuals were not entitled to medical cover. Moreover, under the recent healthcare reforms, insurance providers will no longer perpetuate gender bias in offering medical cover to different groups such as women. In the past, insurance companies could cancel medical coverage or arbitrarily impose charges specifically for women. The recent healthcare reforms have also enabled private insurance to access preventive healthcare services such as disease screening and FDA-approved contraception; unlike in the old healthcare plans in which patients paid for these services out of pocket.

It is also worth noting that the recent healthcare reforms grant low-income individuals financial subsidies pay for their insurance. This has been put in place because healthcare insurance is mandatory for all individuals to enhance access to universal healthcare. It is expected that the recent healthcare reform will enable over 32 million more people who currently lack healthcare insurance to acquire medical coverage through healthcare program expansions and insurance reforms (Jacobs & Skocpol, 2012).

However, the recent healthcare reforms seem to have increased pressure on the U.S healthcare system, especially with regard to primary care practices. Currently, the U.S public healthcare facilities are faced with unprecedented inadequacy due to the ever increasing healthcare demands by the U.S population. Healthcare resources are relatively limited; thus, access to medical services is somehow impaired. Therefore, creating universal access to

11

healthcare from public healthcare facilities might be accompanied by substandard service provision; although the recent reforms incorporate private healthcare providers in facilitating universal access to healthcare.

Impact of Healthcare Policy Changes to Utilization

On the other hand, change to access of healthcare services may influence utilization in different ways. For instance, improved access to healthcare may restore patient satisfaction with public healthcare institutions; since there will be unlimited access to medical services. In the past, most individuals had turned to private healthcare providers since they were believed to offer high-quality services to their clients despite the high costs of treatment. It was observed that most individuals were attracted to private healthcare providers by the reliability and the quality of customer treatment by private healthcare providers. For instance, most private healthcare providers seem to have adopted modern technologies in providing healthcare services to their clients. In contrast, public healthcare providers are reluctant to adopt modern technological approaches which guarantee efficiency and customer satisfaction because some of them are costly.

In retrospect, changes to healthcare access may influence utilization of healthcare facilities in a negative way, especially the public healthcare institutions. It is believed that universal access to healthcare will create the need for high quality services in the public healthcare facilities. As a result, there will be increased competition for services by all individuals seeking medical services, and this situation may cause pressure on the healthcare professionals. The ultimate result for this may be patients' dissatisfaction with public healthcare providers, leading to low turnout of medical service seekers within public healthcare facilities.

Policy Counter: Alternative Policy to ObamaCare

ObamaCare has introduced a single-payer healthcare system in which citizens perceive it as an egalitarian approach. As such, citizens will be receiving healthcare services as a right but not necessarily a basic requirement in life which deserves personal responsibilities. Therefore, it encompasses diverse differences from the free-market healthcare system which has been in use for decades. It is argued that ObamaCare is not ideal for solving the grave problems which have been challenging sustainability of the U.S healthcare system. Levin and Ponnuru (2013) claim "It has consisted chiefly of massive and inefficient entitlements that threaten to bankrupt the nation; the lopsided tax treatment of employer-provided coverage that creates incentives for waste and overspending; and an underdeveloped individual market struggling to fill the gaps" (par. 4).

Therefore, a conservative alternative to ObamaCare involves universal tax benefit for health insurance coverage. This will enhance competition among insurance providers; thus, making insurance cheaper than it was in the earlier system where access to coverage was an enormous challenge. It will also make employees cost-conscious through a tax break which serves as a refundable credit, in which Medicaid operates as a means-based addition to the refundable credit. That way, the middle and low-income Americans can purchase insurance coverage, more or less the same as the high-income individuals, from the same insurance market (Levin & Ponnuru, 2013). It is reported "the new alternative would not require the mandates, taxes and heavy-handed regulations of ObamaCare" (Levin & Ponnuru, 2013 par. 12).

Discussion

In general, the two policy strategies share some commonalities in the sense that they will enhance access to healthcare by all individuals regardless of the socioeconomic status. For instance, ObamaCare aims at extending healthcare insurance benefits to the poor Americans who are not insured. It is estimated that about 49 million Americans lack health insurance while

Government-funded programs coverage benefits only some groups in society. On the other hand, employer-funded insurance coverage is characterized with high insurance premiums which burden the U.S workforce with financial challenges. Moreover, the market purchase of insurance coverage is influenced by the aspects of the free-market economy; thus, making them unaffordable for the low-income population and this is responsible for the high number of uninsured Americans.

However, the universal healthcare policy differs significantly from the alternative policy on the aspect of costs and utilization. In reality, ObamaCare involves huge costs compared to its alternative, and that is why political critics suggest the adoption of the conservative policy alternative which reduces waste and overspending through incentives offered by ObamaCare.

Currently, the healthcare law seems to be facing enormous challenges including its chaotic launch and low first-month enrollment owing to its political connections. Brownstein (2013) states "the administration has now added derision over the law's execution to suspicion about its motivation. In fairness, the health care law, which reported modest but not horrific first-month enrollment numbers, is not the first social program to stumble out of the gate" (par. 4).

Conclusion

In a brief conclusion, ObamaCare seems to have created a single-payer healthcare system, in which risk is shared between the federal governments and the public. The concept of universal healthcare has extended health insurance benefits to middle and low-income individuals who were not insured under the Medicaid policy. In addition, it has extended health benefits to children and youth because it does not have age barriers to reduce health inequalities among the U.S population. In the old system, some social groups were excluded from health insurance coverage, especially the poor who could not afford insurance premiums in the free-market situation. As a result, most of them remained uninsured, and this was attributable to the unsustainability of the U.S healthcare system. Moreover, the healthcare reforms have initiated prominent service provision to patients in public healthcare institutions in an effort of attaining the core objective of quality and affordable healthcare for all individuals. Above all, Federal funding to the healthcare system has been increased to relieve patients of the high cost of treatment (AMSA, 2013).

Despite the benefits of the current healthcare reforms introduced by ObamaCare, the law has attracted immense criticism from the political arena, as well as the U.S public, especially the high-income individuals who are considered to be the losers. In regard to political narrative strategies, high-income individuals who were survived under Medicaid are the losers under ObamaCare while the middle and low-income individuals are the winners. However, the latter were disadvantaged under the Medicaid policy, and this explains why most of them were uninsured.

Therefore, it is believed that a conservative alternative policy to ObamaCare which will transform Medicaid into a refundable credit will solve the grave problems in the U.S healthcare.

References

AMSA(2013). *AMSA Medicaid Expansion Fact Sheet.* Retrieved from http://www.amsa.org/AMSA/Libraries/Initiative_Docs/AMSAMedicaidExpansionFactsh eet.sflb.ashx

APHA (2012). *The Affordable Care Act: The "Individual Mandate" And Other Coverage Provisions.* Retrieved from http://www.apha.org/NR/rdonlyres/C69859CF-F012-4D52-BF52-8F6DAA68C431/0/ACAfactsheetJune2012CoverageProvisions.pdf

Blumberg, L., et.al. (2012). Why Employers will continue to Provide Health Insurance: The Impact of the Affordable Care Act. *Inquiry,* 49(2): 116-26. Retrieved from http://www.ncbi.nlm.nih.gov/pubmed/22931019

Brownstein, R. (2013). *Political Connections: Obamacare's Problems Could Haunt Democrats for Years.* Retrieved from http://www.nationaljournal.com/political-connections/obamacare-s-problems-could-haunt-democrats-for-years-20131115

Carmen, D., Proctor, B. & Smith, J. (2012). *Income, Poverty, and Health Insurance Coverage in the United States: 2011.* Retrieved from http://www.census.gov/prod/2012pubs/p60-243.pdf

Cohen, A. B. (2012). The Debate Over Health Care Rationing: Deja Vu All Over Again? *Inquiry,* 49(2): 90-100. Retrieved from http://www.inquiryjournalonline.org/doi/abs/10.5034/inquiryjrnl_49.02.06

Cudney, A. E. (2002). Providing High-Quality Healthcare: Are We Up To the Task? (Quality and Safety). *Journal of Healthcare Management,* 47(2): 77-80. Retrieved from http://www.emeraldinsight.com/bibliographic_databases.htm?id=1357879&PHPSESSID =p81sb72s0fmmq459h6gego6004

Goody, B., Mentnech, R., & Riley, G. (2002). Changing Nature of Public and Private Health Insurance. *Health Care Financing Review*, 23(3): 1-6. Retrieved from http://www.cms.gov/Research-Statistics-Data-and-Systems/Research/HealthCareFinancingReview/downloads/02Springpg1.pdf

Gorin, H. & Moniz, C. (2012). Medicaid and the Affordable Care Act after the Supreme Court Decision. *Health and Social Work*, 37(4): 195-196. Retrieved from http://hsw.oxfordjournals.org/content/37/4/195.short

GPO (2009). *Congressional Record — Senate.* Retrieved from http://www.gpo.gov/fdsys/pkg/CREC-2009-12-14/pdf/CREC-2009-12-14-pt1-PgS13201-4.pdf#page=1

HHS (2009). *In the Senate of the United States: Affordable Care Act.* Retried from http://www.hhs.gov/healthcare/rights/law/patient-protection.pdf

Jacobs, L. & Skocpol, T. (2012). *Health Care Reform and American Politics: What Everyone Needs to Know, Revised and Updated Edition.* New York, NY: Oxford University Press.

Levin, Y. & Ponnuru, R. (2013). *A Conservative Alternative to ObamaCare.* Retrieved from http://www.eppc.org/publications/a-conservative-alternative-to-obamacare/

Record, L. (2012). Litigating the ACA: Securing the Right to Health within a Framework of Negative Rights. *American Journal of Law & Medicine*, 38 (2/3): 537-547.

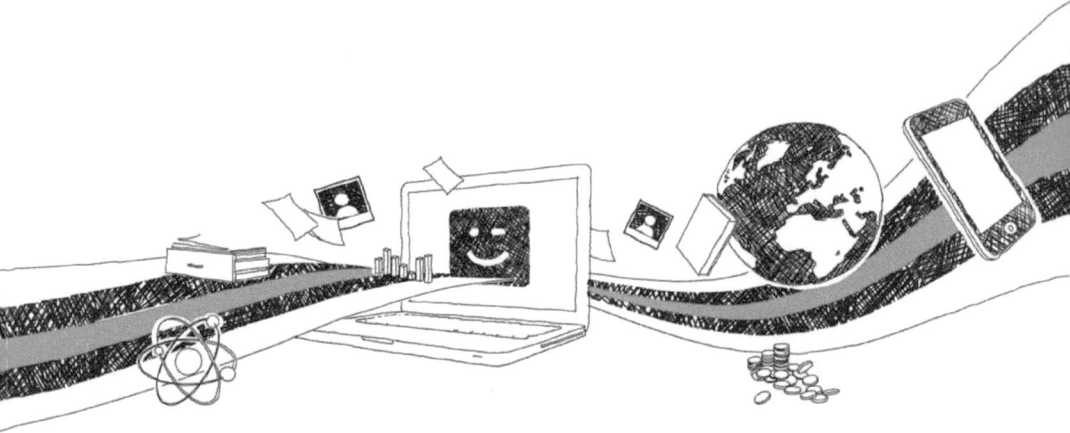
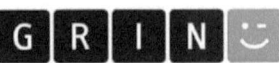